Guillain-Barre Syndrome

Diagnosis, Symptoms, Treatment, Causes,
Doctors, Autoimmune Disorders, Prognosis,
Research, History, and More!

By Frederick Earlstein

Foreword

Autoimmune diseases occur when the immune system starts to mistakenly attack healthy cells and tissues in the body. There are many different autoimmune conditions out there but one of the most devastating is Guillain-Barre syndrome. This disease occurs when the autoimmune system starts to attack the peripheral nervous system, causing weakness and eventual paralysis. Unfortunately, there is no cure for this disease but there are some ways to manage it.

If you or a loved one suffers from Guillain-Barre syndrome you should do yourself a favor and learn everything you can about the condition. That is where this book comes in! In this book you will receive a detailed overview of Guillain-Barre syndrome including its symptoms, causes, and related complications as well as risk factors and treatment options. The more you know about this condition, the better you will be able to fight back against it.

Table of Contents

Introduction

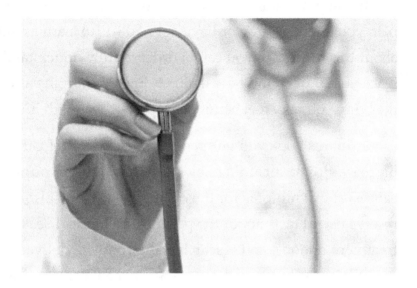

Guillain-Barre syndrome is a rare disorder that occurs when the immune system starts to attack the body's peripheral nervous system. This disease is one of many autoimmune diseases that are still poorly understood by doctors and researchers which is what makes it so difficult to diagnose and to deal with. Unfortunately there is no cure for this disease but there are a number of treatment options which can help a person to manage and cope with their Guillain-Barre syndrome.

If you suffer from Guillain-Barre syndrome you may feel as though you have no control over your own body or over your symptoms. Living with an autoimmune disease can be very difficult and draining, both physically and emotionally. What may help – in addition to the treatment plan you and your doctor have devised – is to learn as much about this disease as you can in order to fully understand it. Once you understand how Guillain-Barre syndrome affects the body you may feel better equipped to deal with it.

In this book you will receive an overview of Guillain-Barre syndrome including key information about the onset, causes, and symptoms for the condition. You will also receive useful facts about the progression of the disease, treatment options, and research being conducted. Even if your Guillain-Barre syndrome is being managed medically, there are certain things you can do that might help to further relive your symptoms. This book includes an overview of dietary changes that may be effective in relieving the symptoms of autoimmune diseases.

By the time you finish this book you will have a deeper understanding of what Guillain-Barre syndrome is and how it affects your body. With this information you can continue to pursue support and management options to improve your quality of life.

Important Terms to Know

Adrenal Gland – the gland responsible for producing the hormones aldosterone, adrenaline, and cortisol.

Albuminocytological Dissociation - an increase in spinal fluid protein concentration without an associated increase in cell count; the key diagnostic abnormality associated with Guillain-Barré Syndrome.

Antibodies – a blood protein produced by the immune system in response to specific antigens; works by combining with the antigen to neutralize the threat.

Antigens - potentially harmful pathogens that enter the body and initiate an immune response.

Areflexia – below normal or absent reflexes; also known as hyporeflexia.

Arrhythmia - irregular heart rhythm.

Ataxia – the loss of control over bodily movements.

Autoimmune Disease - occurs when the immune system starts to attack healthy cells and tissues in addition to the antigens it is supposed to be fighting off.

Autoimmune Protocol (AIP) – a Paleo, gluten-free diet that is designed to address specific problems with inflammation and gastrointestinal damage caused by autoimmune disease.

Central Nervous System - a division of the human nervous system; consists of the brain and spinal cord.

Clinical Trial – a research study that uses human participants to test one or more health-related interventions to evaluate the outcome.

Immunoglobulin – substance belonging to a class of proteins that are found in the serum and cells of the immune system and function as antibodies.

Incontinence - loss of bladder and/or bowel control.

Inflammation – the body's natural response to injury or trauma; long-term, or chronic inflammation is often the result of autoimmune disease.

Leukocytes – white blood cells (WBCs); the active cells of the immune system, work to destroy harmful bacteria, viruses, and other pathogens.

Lymphocytes – a type of leukocyte (white blood cell) that occurs specifically in the lymphatic system; has a single round nucleus.

Myelin Sheath - the coating protecting Schwann cells along the axon between nerves.

Nervous System - the network of organs, muscles, tissues, glands, and nerves which respond to sensory information and produce a response; divided into two parts, the peripheral nervous system and the central nervous system.

Neuropathy – the disease or dysfunction of one or more peripheral nerves; typically results in loss of sensation or muscle weakness.

Paleo Diet – a diet that does not include any foods that would not have been readily available to our Paleolithic-ancestors; excludes grains, legumes, dairy products, artificial sweeteners and processed foods.

Peripheral Nervous System – a division of the human nervous system; consists of sensory neurons and motor neurons.

Plasmapheresis – a treatment involving removing blood plasma from the body through withdrawal of blood and separating it into cells and plasma; the cells are then transfused back into the blood stream.

Respiratory Arrest - the cessation or normal breathing due to improper function of the lungs and breathing muscles.

Chapter One: What is Guillain-Barre Syndrome?

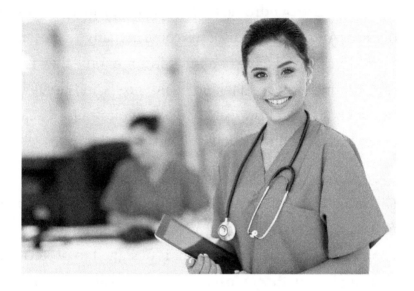

As you may already know, Guillain-Barré Syndrome is a condition where the body's own immune system starts to attack the peripheral nervous system. This condition is fairly rare and doctors still do not understand exactly what causes it, but there are some viable treatment options. Before you can understand the treatment options for this condition, however, you need to understand what it is and how it affects the body. You will learn all of these things and more in this chapter which will prepare you to better understand the content in the rest of this book.

1. Overview of Guillain-Barre Syndrome

The most important thing you need to understand about Guillain-Barré Syndrome (GBS) is that it is an autoimmune disease. Autoimmune diseases come in many shapes and forms but they all have one thing in common – they result in the immune system attacking healthy cells and tissue in the human body. But how exactly does autoimmune disease occur and what effects does it have on the body?

According to the American Autoimmune Related Diseases Association (AARDA), autoimmune disease in all of its different forms affects as many as 50 million Americans. The immune system is designed to protect the body against pathogenic bacteria and viruses as well as other potentially harmful things that invade the body. When pathogenic materials (called antigens) enters the body, it activates the immune system into producing antibodies. These antibodies are developed to attack a specific antigen. Unfortunately, in the case of autoimmune disease, the immune system starts to attack healthy cells and tissues in addition to the antigens it is supposed to be fighting off.

Autoimmune disease can occur in many different organs and systems throughout the body and each disease can affect one or multiple types of tissue. It is estimated that there are 80 different types of autoimmune disease – or more

– and many of them present with similar symptoms. This being the case, it is sometimes difficult for doctors to make an accurate diagnosis. It generally requires a series of blood tests in order to identify and confirm a diagnosis of autoimmune disease because the symptoms can be misleading in many cases.

Guillain-Barré Syndrome is a specific type of autoimmune disease that affects the peripheral nervous system. The human nervous system is divided into two parts – the peripheral nervous system (PNS) and the central nervous system (CNS). The peripheral nervous system consists of the nerves and ganglia that are located outside the central nervous system – its purpose is to connect the central nervous system to the limbs and organs in the body. Essentially, the peripheral nervous system provides the pathway of sensory and motor neurons which transport communications between the central nervous system and the rest of the body.

In the case of Guillain-Barré Syndrome, the immune system starts to attack the cells and nerves in the peripheral nervous system. This results in a number of different symptoms, most of which are related to sensations and activity of the extremities which can then spread throughout the entire body. The first symptom of Guillain-Barré

Syndrome is often weakness or tingling in the extremities, followed eventually by paralysis.

Unfortunately, the cause of Guillain-Barré Syndrome is unknown and in severe cases, it can be a medical emergency. Most people suffering from this condition need to be hospitalized at some point, especially in cases of total paralysis. When the body becomes paralyzed, the person may have difficulty breathing and the paralysis can also affect the heart rate and blood pressure. Even in severe cases like this, however, recovery is possible. There is no cure for Guillain-Barré Syndrome but the symptoms and progression can be managed with medications and certain therapies. Specific dietary changes may also help to reduce autoimmune activity which can slow the disease.

2. History of the Disease

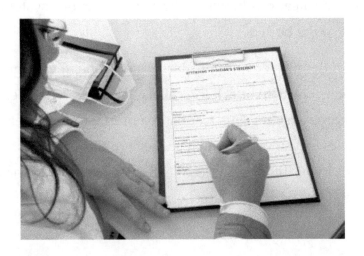

The disease now known as Guillain-Barré Syndrome was first described by a French physician named Jean-Baptiste Octave Landry in 1859. It wasn't until 1916, however, that the key diagnostic abnormality associated with the disease - albuminocytological dissociation, or an increase in spinal fluid protein concentration without an associated increase in cell count – was described. This description was made by Georges Guillain, Jean Alexandre Barré, and Andre Strohl. The description was made when these physicians diagnosed two soldiers with the condition.

In 1951, a British neurologist by the name of Edwin Bickerstaff described a variant of the disease which involved brainstem encephalitis and, in 1956 a Canadian neurologist by the name of C. Miller Fisher described another variant of the disease. Though these variants were briefly mentioned in the report written by Georges Guillain, they were not fully described until 1938. Since this time, other subtypes of Guillain-Barré Syndrome have been described such as an axonal subtype, one type causing pharyngeal-cervical-brachial weakness, and another causing pure ataxia.

Though the various forms of Guillain-Barré Syndrome were described during the 1930s, it wasn't until the 1970s that diagnostic criteria for the disease were developed. This development occurred following a series of cases that were linked to the swine flu vaccine. The diagnostic criteria were refined in 1990 and the case definition for the disease was revised in 2009 by the Brighton Collaboration for the sake of vaccine safety. The first use of plasma exchange for the treatment of Guillain-Barré Syndrome occurred in 1978 and the use of intravenous immunoglobulin was first introduced in 1988.

3. Other Common Autoimmune Diseases

As you have already learned, there are as many as 80 different types of autoimmune disease, or more. While each condition is unique, the symptoms of many autoimmune diseases tend to overlap. Unfortunately, many of the symptoms associated with autoimmune disease also overlap with symptoms of other diseases. For this reason, many people who have autoimmune disease do not even know it. <u>There are, however, some common signs to look for when it comes to autoimmune disease</u>:

- Muscle spasms, tremors, weakness and joint pain.
- Sensitivity to sunlight, recurrent rashes, or hives.
- Unexplained weight loss or weight gain.
- Difficulty focusing and concentrating.
- Chronic fatigue and problems with insomnia.
- White patches of skin and/or hair loss.
- Blood or mucus in the stool or diarrhea.

- Dry mouth, skin or eyes.
- Tingling or numbness in the hands and feet.
- Blood clotting issues or multiple miscarriages.

What many people do not realize is that if you have an autoimmune disease, your risk for developing a second one is much higher than the risk for the average person. In many cases, autoimmune diseases fluctuate between periods of remission and flare-ups, though they can never be fully cured. This is why treatment options for autoimmune disease are typically aimed toward relieving symptoms – a cure is not possible.

Not only can your risk for developing autoimmune disease increase if you already have one, but there are other factors which affect your risk as well. For example, about 75% of people affected by autoimmune disease are women – autoimmune diseases also have a genetic factor so if a member of your family has one, your risk may be greater. The AARDA also states that certain ethnicities including Hispanics, African Americans, and Native Americans have a higher risk for autoimmune disease.

Autoimmune diseases come in all shapes and sizes but some of them are more common than others. Below you will find a list of some of the most common autoimmune diseases according to the AARDA:

- **Celiac Sprue Disease** – triggered by consumption of gluten (a protein found in wheat, barley, and rye) which causes damage to the lining of the small intestine
- **Rheumatoid Arthritis** – painful inflammation of the joints and surrounding tissues
- **Pernicious Anemia** – a decrease in red blood cell count caused by an inability to absorb the vitamin B12 (cobalamin)
- **Systemic Lupus Erythematosus** – a condition that affects the function of the kidneys, brain, and other organs as well as the skin and joints
- **Vitiligo** – causes white patches to form in the skin caused by a loss of pigment
- **Psoriasis** – a skin condition that results in redness and irritation as well as the formation of flaky patches
- **Inflammatory Bowel Disease** – a group of inflammatory diseases affecting the small intestine and colon
- **Hashimoto's Disease** – chronic inflammation of the thyroid gland which interferes with the production of thyroid hormones
- **Graves' Disease** – a condition characterized by an overactive thyroid

- **Addison's Disease** – a condition that results in the insufficient production and utilization of adrenal hormones

Unfortunately, the cause of autoimmune disease is unknown though there is some evidence to suggest that certain things like bacteria, viruses, drugs, and various environmental or chemical irritants can be a trigger. In order to diagnose autoimmune disease you may be subjected to various blood tests as well as a medical and family history. Later in this book you will learn the specifics about diagnosing autoimmune disease as it relates to Guillain-Barré Syndrome in particular.

Chapter Two: Signs and Symptoms

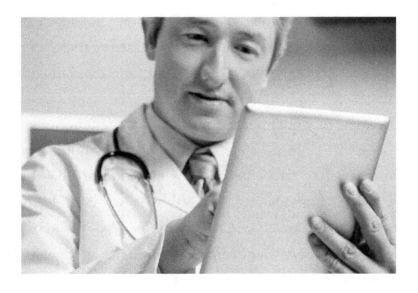

Now that you have a better understanding of what Guillain-Barré Syndrome is, you have a foundation of knowledge on which to base your understanding of the symptoms, onset, and progression of the disease. In this chapter you will learn about the clinical presentations of the disease as well as some key information about how the disease manifests and how it progresses. Learning this information will help you to better understand the content of the next chapter which covers the potential causes of Guillain-Barré Syndrome as well as the mechanism of the disease and the various subtypes.

1. *Common Signs and Symptoms*

As you have already learned, autoimmune diseases like Guillain-Barré Syndrome can sometimes be tricky to diagnose because many of the symptoms overlap with other diseases. At a certain point, however, the symptoms of GBS become very obvious and medical treatment becomes a necessity. Unfortunately, by the time the symptoms become obvious they can be very severe and widespread – they can also be life threatening. This is why it is a good idea to familiarize yourself with the common signs and symptoms of Guillain-Barré Syndrome so you do not let it get to that point before you seek treatment.

In most cases, Guillain-Barré Syndrome presents with tingling and weakness in the extremities – particularly the feet and legs. The tingling sensations may then spread into the upper body and down the arms. Many people describe the sensation as prickling, like pins and needles. The sensation is usually strongest in the fingers, toes, wrists, and ankles, though about 10% of people with GBS experience symptoms that begin in the face or in the hands and arms.

As Guillain-Barré Syndrome progresses, symptoms may spread into the upper body and deeper into the muscles and connective tissues. This may result in increased weakness in the legs which can cause difficulty walking and an inability to climb stairs. Many patients also experience difficulty with facial movements such as chewing, speaking, and swallowing. If the disease is allowed to progress, this may worsen to the point where the person experiences difficulty breathing.

Some people with Guillain-Barré Syndrome experience severe muscle pains that feel like cramps and worsen at night. Eventually, this disease can lead to loss of bladder or bowel control (incontinence). In some cases, patients experience rapid heart rate and changes in blood pressure. For most Guillain-Barré Syndrome patients, the symptoms reach their height about two to four weeks after the initial presentation. Once the symptoms plateau, many people begin to recover after another two to four weeks with proper treatment.

2. Onset and Progression of the Disease

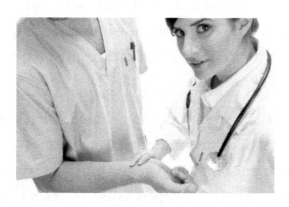

In many cases, the symptoms of Guillain-Barré Syndrome come on gradually but once initial symptoms present, the disease has the potential to progress very rapidly. For some people, symptoms can become serious – even life-threatening – within a matter of hours. On average, symptoms increase in severity over the course of 12 hours up to two weeks, though 1 in 5 people may experience worsening symptoms over a period of up to four weeks or more.

After the symptoms have plateaued (reached their maximum level of severity), they may persist at a consistent level for some time – this phase can last anywhere from two days to six months. The most common length for the plateau phase is about one week. During this phase, about one third of Guillain-Barré Syndrome patients retain their ability to walk and about 50% of patients experience involvement of the cranial nerves which affect the muscles in the head and face. More than half of all Guillain-Barré Syndrome patients also experience pain-related symptoms during this phase such as painful tingling, back pain, muscle pain, and pain in the head or neck.

About 25% of all people diagnosed with Guillain-Barré Syndrome develop some degree of weakness in the breathing muscles which leads to respiratory failure, the inability to breathe independently. In many cases, this condition is complicated by secondary infections like pneumonia or by blood clots in the lungs and/or bleeding in the digestive tract. This happens in about 60% of patients who receive artificial ventilation.

About two-thirds of people diagnosed with Guillain-Barré Syndrome also experience autonomic or involuntary nervous system involvement. The severity of involvement may vary with about 20% of cases showing severe fluctuations in blood pressure as well as irregular heartbeat. In some cases, the heart actually stops beating - cases like this may require the implantation of a pacemaker. Other potential problems associated with this type of involvement includes abnormal perspiration and changes in the normal reactivity of the pupil. This type of involvement can occur even in GBS patients who are not experiencing severe muscle weakness.

Chapter Three: Causes of the Disease

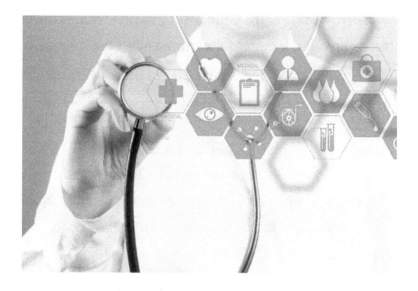

One of the biggest problems with Guillain-Barré Syndrome is the fact that it is tricky to diagnose. It is also unfortunate that the exact cause of the disease is unknown – this affects the efficacy of treatment options. Though there is no single cause for Guillain-Barré Syndrome, scientists and researchers have confirmed correlations with the syndrome and various infections and other risk factors. In this chapter you will learn about the potential causes for this disease as well as information about the mechanism for the disease and various subtypes that have been identified.

1. What Causes Guillain-Barre Syndrome?

The exact cause of Guillain-Barré Syndrome is unknown but out of all the people diagnosed with the disease, about two-thirds have experienced some type of infection 3 to 6 weeks prior to the onset of symptoms. The most common infections seen in cases like this are respiratory tract infection or gastroenteritis. In some cases, the exact nature of the prior infection can accurately be identified. In about 30% of cases, the infection is caused by *Campylobacter jejuni* bacteria and, in 10% of cases, the cause of infection is the cytomegalovirus (HHV-5).

Though these infections have been linked to many cases of active Guillain-Barré Syndrome, a relatively small number of people who experience these infections ever develop the disease. In fact, the incidence of *Campylobacter jejuni* infections which result in GBS is only about 0.25 to 0.65 per 1,000 cases. In cases involving the cytomegalovirus, only 0.6 to 2.2 cases progress to Guillain-Barré Syndrome out of every 1,000. Scientists and researchers have reason to believe that some strains of *Campylobacter jejuni* bacteria are more likely to contribute to the development of GBS than are some others.

Though these two infections are correlated with GBS in the highest number of cases, links have been forged with other infections as well. For example, two types of herpes virus – varicella zoster/HHV-3 and Epstein-Barr virus/HHV-4) – have been associated with Guillain-Barré Syndrome in some cases. It has also been discovered that previous hepatitis E infections are fairly common in patients diagnosed with GBS.

During the 1970s, several cases of Guillain-Barré Syndrome were linked to the influenza vaccine that was developed to protect against swine flu. The Institute of Medicine conducted a thorough study and found that the increased risk for GBS was about 1 additional case per 100,000 people who received the vaccine. The link between the 1976 swine flu vaccine and increased risk for GBS was reviewed in depth in 2003 but the link between GBS and flu vaccines from other years is unclear.

Though flu vaccines may play a role in triggering Guillain-Barré Syndrome in rare cases, scientists believe that it is more likely for someone to develop GBS following a flu infection than the vaccine. Surgery has been known to trigger Guillain-Barré Syndrome in rare cases as well. As for genetic or environmental risk factors, GBS has not been seen to affect individuals of any age or sex more than others. People of any age can develop the disease and it seems to affect men and women equally.

2. *Mechanism of the Disease*

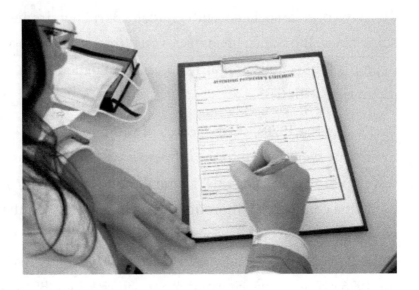

You already know that Guillain-Barré Syndrome is the result of autoimmune activity that attacks the nerve cells, particularly the nerve cells of the peripheral nervous system. In order to truly understand this disease, however, you need to know what kind of changes it causes to occur in the body. The nerve cells located in the spinal cord have a body which is called the soma. Each nerve also has a projection, or arm, that is called an axon and it serves to carry electrical impulses to the various muscles in the body. These axons are protected by a myelin sheath which is made up of Schwann cells.

Along the length of each axon, there are certain areas between the Shwann cells where some of the axon is exposed. Various subtypes of Guillain-Barré Syndrome attack the axon in these gaps. For example, the demyelinating variant of GBS causes damage to the myelin sheath protecting the axon – this damage is facilitated by white blood cells called lymphocytes. The axonal variant of GBS involves IgG antibodies which can damage the myelin sheath without the involvement of any lymphocytes.

In all autoimmune diseases, antibodies are what causes the damage – they are intended to attack pathogenic materials that enter the body but they end up attacking the body's own cells and tissues as well. Several different types of antibodies have been identified in cases of Guillain-Barré Syndrome. In the axonal subtype of the disease, antibodies have been known to bind with gangliosides such as GM1, GD1a, GQ1b, and GT1a. Certain gangliosides are linked to specific variants of the disease.

3. Subtypes of Guillain-Barre Syndrome

Guillain-Barré Syndrome can produce a wide variety of different symptoms and different groups of symptoms are associated with particular variants, or subtypes of the disease. This makes diagnosing GBS something of a challenge, especially since all of the different subtypes also have partial forms. It is also worth noting that the different subtypes of GBS involve different antibodies. <u>Below you will find an overview of the six most common subtypes of Guillain-Barré Syndrome</u>:

Acute Inflammatory Demyelinating Polyneuropathy (AIDP) – This subtype is most commonly seen in North America and Europe, causing symptoms which may include muscle weakness, tingling sensations, and frequent cranial nerve weakness as well as autonomic involvement.

Acute Motor Axonal Neuropathy (AMAN) – This subtype is most common in Asia as well as Central and South America – it is sometimes nicknamed "Chinese paralytic syndrome". Common symtpoms include isolated muscle weakness without any sensory symptoms in under 10% of cases – cranial nerve involvement is uncommon.

Acute Motor and Sensory Axonal Neuropathy (AMSAN) – This subtype causes severe muscle weakness similar to the AMAN subtype but with the addition of sensory loss.

Axonal Polyneuropathy with Reduced or Absent Sensory Action Potential – This subtype may cause muscle weakness with a reduction or loss in sensory action potential. It may also involve gangliosides against the antibodies GM1 and GD1a.

Pharyngeal-Cervical-Brachial Variant – This subtype typically causes weakness in the throat muscles as well as in the face, neck, and shoulders.

Miller Fisher Syndrome - This variant is more common in men than in women at a 2-to-1 ratio and the average age of onset is 43 years old. This type causes ataxia as well as eye muscle weakness and areflexia, usually without any evidence of limb weakness.

Chapter Four: Diagnosis and Prognosis

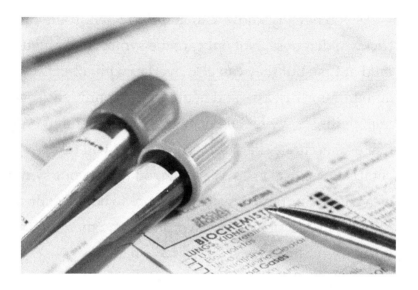

By now it should be clear to you that Guillain-Barré Syndrome can be very serious. As serious as this disease can be in many cases, it is still somewhat difficult to diagnose until the symptoms have become very severe. In this chapter you will learn about the different tests that can be used to diagnose GBS and you will receive some key information regarding the prognosis for Guillain-Barré Syndrome patients. You will also receive information about the potential complications that have been associated with Guillain-Barré Syndrome in some cases.

1. Diagnosis of Guillain-Barre Syndrome

As you already know, Guillain-Barré Syndrome can be tricky to diagnose. Not only are the symptoms sometimes mild at first, but they can also overlap with other autoimmune diseases and neurological conditions such as meningitis, heavy metal poisoning, or botulism. In order to make an accurate diagnosis, your doctor will take a complete medical history, asking you about your symptoms as well as your family history. Be sure to be as detailed as possible in describing your symptoms and mention any infections or illnesses you may have had.

<u>In addition to a medical and family history, your doctor may also administer certain tests including the following:</u>

- **Spinal Tap (Lumbar Puncture)** – In this test, a small amount of spinal fluid is taken from the spinal canal via needle and then tested.

- **Electromyography** – For this test, your doctor will insert thin-needle electrodes into your muscles to measure nerve activity.

- **Nerve Conduction Study** – In this test, electrodes are taped to your skin over the nerves and a small shock is passed through them to test the speed of nerve signals.

In addition to these tests, your doctor may also require certain blood tests to check for autoimmune activity. In most cases, however, blood tests are performed to rule out other potential medical causes for your symptoms such as low potassium levels. It may also happen that your doctor wants to have an MRI of the spinal cord performed to confirm Guillain-Barré Syndrome as the cause for muscle weakness, ruling out other potential causes such as spinal cord compression or herniated disc.

2. Prognosis for the Disease

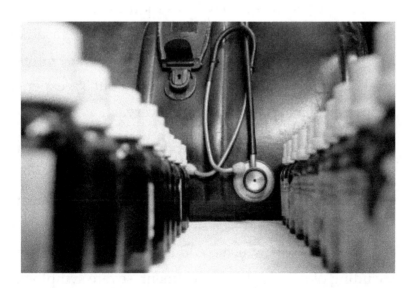

Unfortunately, Guillain-Barré Syndrome has the potential to be very serious and symptoms can develop and progress very quickly in some cases. It is also worth noting that recovery from this disease is rarely quick. As you may remember from an earlier section, most patients experience a worsening of symptoms that lasts anywhere from half a day to two weeks – it can even last as long as four weeks in some cases.

Once the symptoms reach the peak of severity, most patients go through a plateau period where symptoms stabilize for days, weeks, or months on end. The average length of the plateau period for Guillain-Barré Syndrome patients is about 1 week. After the plateau period comes the recovery period which may be as short as several weeks or as long as several years – it is different in every case. About 30% of GBS patients still experience some degree of residual weakness after 3 years of recovery and bout 3% experience a relapse even many years after recovery.

According to the Mayo Clinic, about 80% of Guillain-Barré Syndrome patients regain their ability to walk independently after 6 months and about 60% of patients regain their former muscle strength. Unfortunately, there are certain risk factors which could lead to a worse prognosis including old age, delay of treatment, severe symptoms or rapid progression, and the prolonged use of a respirator device. It is also worth noting that many GBS patients experience psychological as well as physical problems that come with changes in mobility and decreased independence.

3. Complications of Guillain-Barre Syndrome

Guillain-Barré Syndrome is a disease that affects the peripheral nervous system which means that it can interfere with the communications between your nerves and your muscles. When the nerves begin to break down and malfunction it can lead to a number of serious complications. <u>Below you will find an overview of some of the most common complications that have been associated with Guillain-Barré Syndrome</u>:

Breathing Problems – When weakness and paralysis caused by GBS spreads to the respiratory muscles it can lead to fatal respiratory arrest. About 30% of patients diagnosed with GBS will need artificial respiration at some point during their course of treatment.

Loss of Sensation – While many people with Guillain-Barré Syndrome recover completely, some are left with residual loss of sensation or numbness – some also experience minor tingling or muscle weakness.

Heart Problems – Some of the most serious side effects of GBS are fluctuations in blood pressure and irregular heart rhythm (arrhythmia).

Nerve Pain – As many as 50% of Guillain-Barré Syndrome patients experience some level of nerve pain and it can be quite severe - in most cases it can be managed with pain medications.

Incontinence – Guillain-Barré Syndrome can lead to sluggish bowel movement and urine retention which can cause reduction or complete loss of bladder and bowel control.

Blood Clots – When Guillain-Barré Syndrome results in loss of mobility or complete paralysis there is an increased risk for blood clots – taking blood thinners and wearing compression socks may help prevent this.

Bedsores – In cases where GBS leads to immobility, the risk for developing pressure sores (or bedsores) increases. Frequent repositioning during bed rest may help to prevent this complication.

Flare-Ups – As an autoimmune disease, Guillain-Barré Syndrome can fluctuate between periods of remission and flare-ups of symptoms. Approximately 5% of people diagnosed with GBS experience at least one relapse following successful treatment.

In some cases, the symptoms of Guillain-Barré Syndrome are mild and short-lived. It is in cases where symptoms present early and become severe that complications are most likely to occur. In addition to the complications listed above, death is another potential complication that can occur when problems with breathing or heart troubles are also present and severe.

Chapter Five: Treatment Options

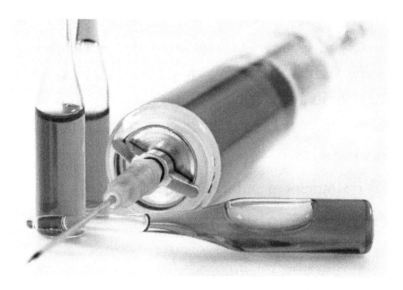

While it is true that Guillain-Barré Syndrome cannot be cured, there are certain treatment options available which can mitigate the severity of symptoms. The treatment options available to a Guillain-Barré Syndrome patient may vary depending on the progression of the disease – different treatments may be required in cases of medical emergency where breathing has been compromised or cardiac function is sub-optimal. You will learn about the various treatment options in this chapter and, in the next chapter, you will receive an introduction to dietary changes that can be supportive for Guillain-Barré Syndrome patients.

1. Overview of Treatment Options

The goal of treatment for Guillain-Barré Syndrome is to lessen the severity of symptoms and to accelerate healing. In some cases, treatment may also have the goal of resolving complications such as respiratory failure or cardiac arrhythmia. <u>The most common treatment options for GBS are listed below</u>:

- Immunoglobulin Therapy
- Plasmapheresis
- Medication
- Physical Therapy
- Hydrotherapy
- Dietary Modifications
- Counselling

In the following pages you will receive more detailed information about each of these treatment methods for Guillain-Barré Syndrome.

2. *Immunoglobulin Therapy*

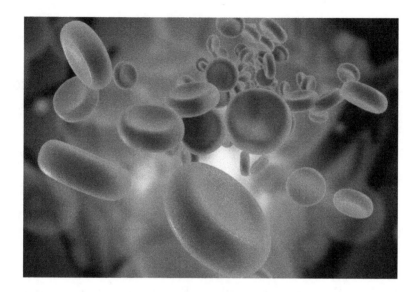

One of the most effective treatments which has been shown to speed recovery for Guillain-Barré Syndrome is immunoglobulin. When large doses of immunoglobulin are given intravenously it has been shown to lessen the duration of Guillain-Barré Syndrome symptoms. This treatment is just as effective as plasmapheresis and it is often preferable because it does not require the use of a large venous catheter.

3. Plasmapheresis (Plasma Exchange)

Probably the most common treatment for Guillain-Barré Syndrome is plasmapheresis. This treatment involves withdrawing blood from the patient and passing it through a series of filters which separate the different types of blood cells and to remove the plasma. The filtered cells are then suspended in synthetic or donor plasma and transfused back into the patient's body. The patients who respond best to this treatment are those that have been diagnosed early in the progression of the disease. This course of treatment is effective in approximately 70% of patients and it can help to reduce the course of Guillain-Barré Syndrome symptoms, provide relief from symptoms, and prevent paralysis from setting in.

4. Medication

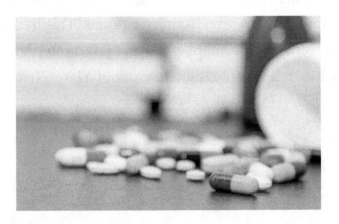

For the most part, medical treatments for Guillain-Barré Syndrome are aimed at providing relief from symptoms such as pain, muscle spasms, and loss of sensation. Joint and muscle pain can be treated with over-the-counter analgesic medications like aspirin. For severe pain, prescription medications like acetaminophen with hydrocodone might be issued.

In some cases, muscle spasms and tremors respond to treatment with relaxants like diazepam and issues with tingling or sensation problems may be managed with anticonvulsants or tricyclic antidepressants. Corticosteroids have also been used to relieve autoimmune symptoms but they have been shown to actually worsen Guillain-Barré Syndrome so they should not be used in this case. There are a few studies currently underway regarding the efficacy of other medical treatments for Guillain-Barré Syndrome.

5. Other Treatment Options

In addition to the conventional treatments already mentioned, there are a few other options for Guillain-Barré Syndrome which may be effective in some cases. For example, some patients respond well to physical therapy treatments during the progressive or plateau phase of the illness. This type of treatment can help to prevent stiffness in the muscles and joints. During the recovery period, many doctors prescribe physical therapy to help the patient regain mobility and muscle strength so they can also regain some of their independence.

Another type of supportive therapy which may be beneficial in some cases is hydrotherapy. Also known as whirlpool therapy, hydrotherapy can help to relieve pain and it may also help patients with severe Guillain-Barré Syndrome regain the mobility and strength of some of their muscles and limbs. There are only a limited number of studies regarding the use of physical therapy for Guillain-Barré Syndrome in terms of long-term relief but it generally helps with short-term recovery.

For patients with respiratory failure or breathing problems, artificial respiration via intubation may be an element of treatment and it is generally administered in a hospital ICU. Many Guillain-Barré Syndrome also benefit from psychotherapy or counselling to help them deal with issues such as loss of mobility and independence. For some patients, paralysis sets in very suddenly and it can be difficult to deal with emotionally as well as physically. Counseling is often a long-term treatment for patients with Guillain-Barré Syndrome.

Chapter Six: Diet for Autoimmune Disease

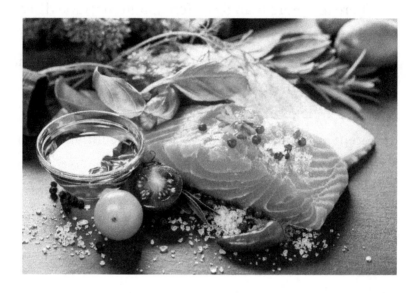

While immunotherapy and medical therapies are the most common treatments for Guillain-Barré Syndrome, there are other options which can provide benefits as well. For example, many people experience relief from autoimmune symptoms when they make specific changes to their diet. In fact, there is a diet called the Autoimmune Protocol (AIP) which is designed specifically for this purpose. In this chapter you will receive an introduction to dietary modifications that benefit Guillain-Barré Syndrome patients as well as detailed information about the Autoimmune Protocol and some tasty recipes.

1. Nutrition and Autoimmune Disease

There are more than 80 different autoimmune diseases out there and each one affects the human body in a different way. What researchers have found, however, is that many autoimmune diseases respond positively to specific dietary changes. One of the most common elements that links different autoimmune diseases is chronic inflammation. Inflammation is the body's natural response to trauma and it is designed to protect the affected area, drawing more blood to the area to speed healing. When inflammation becomes chronic (doesn't go away), however, it can lead to serious problems.

One of the main goals for the Autoimmune Protocol (AIP) is to relieve chronic inflammation. This can be accomplished by increasing your consumption of anti-inflammatory foods – this includes things like fresh fruits and vegetables, omega fatty acids, and lean proteins. It also means reducing your consumption of inflammatory foods like refined carbohydrates, processed sugar, dairy products, alcohol, and gluten.

Another dietary change that can be beneficial for autoimmune diseases like Guillain-Barré Syndrome is increased consumption of Vitamin D, the sunshine vitamin. Numerous studies have shown a link between sunlight exposure and Vitamin D intake with reduced risk for autoimmune disease. There have also been studies to show that people with confirmed autoimmune disease often exhibit Vitamin D deficiencies. Some natural sources of Vitamin D include wild-caught salmon, mushrooms, canned tuna, sardines, mackerel and cod liver oil.

For many people, autoimmune disease causes gastrointestinal problems which can be remedied in part by increasing your consumption of prebiotics and probiotics. Fermented foods, for example, help to boost beneficial bacteria in the digestive system. There are also prebiotic foods like garlic, onions, dandelion greens, and asparagus which can be beneficial. Eating more omega-3 fatty acids can also help with inflammation and autoimmune disease. Natural sources of omega-3 fatty acids include marine fish and fish oils.

In addition to increasing your consumption of certain foods, avoiding some foods may also be beneficial for autoimmune diseases like Guillain-Barré Syndrome. For example, gluten is a common trigger for autoimmune symptoms and it is best avoided. Other studies have shown that dairy products and processed grains can be damaging for autoimmune patients.

2.) *Autoimmune Dietary Protocol*

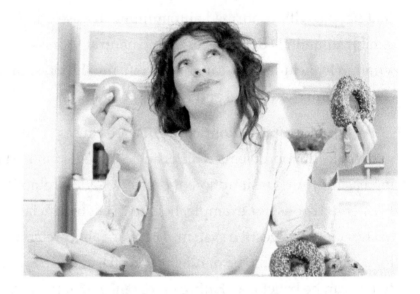

In order to improve your diet as a supportive therapy for your Guillain-Barré Syndrome you do not have to memorize a long list of restricted foods – you can simply follow the template set by the Autoimmune Protocol (AIP). This diet was developed specifically to counteract the effects of autoimmune disease and it may help you to find relief from your symptoms. <u>The basics of the Autoimmune Protocol are listed below</u>:

- Avoid all nuts, seeds, beans and legumes (including spices made from seeds)

- Do not consume grains (even gluten-free grains like rice and corn)
- Avoid processed sugar and artificial sweeteners (such as xylitol and stevia)
- Do not consume eggs, chocolate, or dairy products
- Avoid all processed foods and convenience foods
- Do not eat nightshade vegetables (potatoes, tomatoes, peppers, eggplant, and chilis)
- Choose healthy fats over vegetable oils (choose olive oil, coconut oil, ghee, and avocado)
- Limit your consumption of fruit to 2 pieces a day
- Increase your consumption of fermented foods
- Enjoy vegetables freely (except nightshades)
- Choose lean, grass-fed meats and wild-caught fish
- Drink plenty of green tea, herbal tea, and bone broth
- Use natural sweeteners sparingly (1 teaspoon a day)
- Enjoy fresh herbs and non-seed spices freely

This list may seem exhausting at first or difficult to understand but it is actually quite simple. Do not eat any processed foods, refined grains, or high-glycemic carbohydrates. Avoid dairy products and eggs, including chocolate. Choose healthy fats and oils and limit your consumption of fruit and natural sweeteners. Eat plenty of lean protein – grass-fed or wild-caught, if possible. Enjoy plenty of non-nightshade vegetables and try to eat some fermented foods as well.

3. Autoimmune Diet Sample Recipes

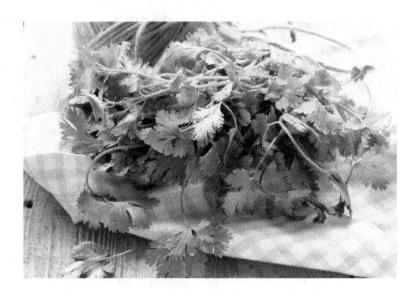

It could take you some time to get used to the Autoimmune Protocol but you will get the hang of it eventually. To help you out, you will find a collection of AIP recipes for breakfast, lunch, dinner, and dessert in this section. Try a few recipes for yourself to see just how simple the AIP can really be if you give it a chance.

Recipes Included in this Chapter:

Cinnamon Zucchini Muffins

Spiced Pumpkin Porridge

Coconut Avocado Lime Smoothie

Triple Berry Mint Smoothie

Chapter Six: Diet for Autoimmune Disease

Apple Sage Breakfast Sausage

Tropical Mango Coconut Smoothie

Honey Coconut Flour Pancakes

Fermented Coconut Yogurt

Baked Coconut Chicken Tenders

Roasted Acorn Squash Soup

Slow Cooker Pulled Pork

Arugula Salad with Apples

Creamy Carrot Ginger Soup

Balsamic Chicken Salad

Chilled Avocado Soup with Lime

Avocado Shrimp Salad

Seared Swordfish w/ Mango Salsa

Rosemary Baked Chicken

Garlic Herb Pork Loin

Lemon Garlic Steamed Mussels

Honey Grilled Salmon Fillets

Beef and Mushroom Stew

Seared Scallops w/ Onions

Lemon Artichoke Zucchini Pasta

Cinnamon Banana Smoothie

Coconut Apple Crisp

Baked Squash Fries

Cucumber Melon Smoothie

Easy Coconut Flour Cookies

Homemade Apple Fruit Leather

Vanilla Coconut Milk Ice Cream

Salted Baked Zucchini Chips

Breakfast Recipes

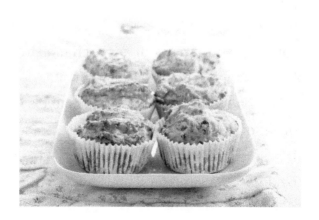

Cinnamon Zucchini Muffins

Servings: 12

Ingredients:

- 1 ½ cups fresh shredded zucchini
- 1/3 cup plain gelatin
- 1/3 cup warm water
- ½ cup pure maple syrup
- ¼ cup melted coconut oil
- 2 teaspoons vanilla extract
- ¾ cups coconut flour
- 2 teaspoons ground cinnamon
- 1 teaspoon baking soda
- ½ teaspoon salt

Instructions:

1. Preheat the oven to 350°F and line a regular muffin pan with paper liners.
2. Spread the shredded zucchini on a clean towel then roll it up and wring out as much moisture as possible.
3. Whisk together the gelatin and water in a medium mixing bowl then whisk in the maple syrup, coconut oil, and vanilla extract.
4. In a separate bowl, stir together the coconut flour, baking soda, cinnamon and salt.

5. Stir the dry ingredients into the wet until smooth then fold in the shredded zucchini.
6. Spoon the mixture into the muffin pan, filling each cup no more than ¾ full.
7. Bake for 24 to 28 minutes until a knife inserted in the center comes out clean.
8. Cool the muffins for 5 minutes in the pan then turn out onto a wire rack to cool completely.

Coconut Avocado Lime Smoothie

Servings: 2

Ingredients:

- 1 medium frozen banana, peeled and chopped
- ½ ripe avocado, pitted and chopped
- 1 cup canned coconut milk
- ½ cup ice cubes
- 2 tablespoons fresh lime juice
- 1 teaspoon fresh lime zest
- 1 teaspoon raw honey

Instructions:

1. Combine all of the ingredients in a high-speed blender.
2. Pulse several times to chop the ingredients.

3. Blend on high speed for 30 to 60 seconds until smooth.

4. Pour into glasses and enjoy immediately.

Spiced Pumpkin Porridge

Servings: 6

Ingredients:

- 1 tablespoon coconut oil
- ¾ cups canned coconut milk
- 1 (15-ounce) can pumpkin puree
- 1 teaspoon ground cinnamon
- 2 tablespoons plain gelatin
- 2 tablespoons warm water
- ½ cup coconut flour
- 1 tablespoon maple syrup

Instructions:

1. Heat the coconut oil in a medium saucepan over medium heat.
2. Whisk in the coconut milk, pumpkin, and cinnamon.
3. In a separate bowl, whisk together the gelatin and water.
4. Whisk the gelatin mixture into the coconut milk mixture and whisk in the coconut flour.

5. Let the mixture simmer for 4 to 5 minutes until thick then stir in the maple syrup.

6. Cook 1 minute more then spoon into bowls to serve.

Triple Berry Mint Smoothie

Servings: 2

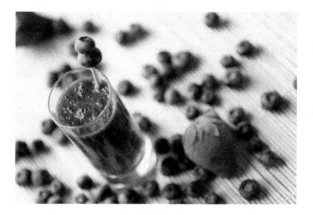

Ingredients:

- 1 ½ cups frozen blueberries
- 1 cup frozen sliced strawberries
- ½ cup frozen raspberries
- 1 cup coconut water, chilled
- ½ cup fresh squeezed orange juice
- ¼ cup fresh chopped mint

Instructions:

1. Combine all of the ingredients in a high-speed blender.

2. Pulse several times to chop the ingredients.

3. Blend on high speed for 30 to 60 seconds until smooth.

4. Pour into glasses and enjoy immediately.

Apple Sage Breakfast Sausage

Servings: 6

Ingredients:

- 1 tablespoon coconut oil
- 1 medium yellow onion, chopped
- 1 Granny smith apple, peeled, cored, and diced
- ½ inch fresh grated ginger
- 2 cloves minced garlic
- 1 teaspoon dried sage
- Salt and pepper to taste
- 2 pounds grass-fed ground pork
- ½ tablespoon cider vinegar
- Honey to taste

Instructions:

1. Preheat the oven to 350°F and line a baking sheet with parchment.

2. Melt the coconut oil in a large skillet over medium-high heat.

3. Add the onions, apples, ginger, garlic and sage then season with salt and pepper to taste.
4. Cook for 5 to 6 minutes then transfer the mixture to a food processor.
5. Blend the mixture until smooth then add the remaining ingredients.
6. Pulse the mixture until it comes together then shape it into small patties by hand.
7. Place the patties on the baking sheet and bake for 25 to 30 minutes until cooked through.

Tropical Mango Coconut Smoothie
Servings: 2

Ingredients:

- 1 cup frozen chopped mango
- 1 cup frozen chopped pineapple
- 1 small frozen banana, peeled and chopped
- 1 cup canned coconut milk
- ½ cup ice cubes
- ¼ cup fresh squeezed orange juice
- 1 teaspoon raw honey

Instructions:

1. Combine all of the ingredients in a high-speed blender.
2. Pulse several times to chop the ingredients.

3. Blend on high speed for 30 to 60 seconds until smooth.

4. Pour into glasses and enjoy immediately.

Honey Coconut Flour Pancakes

Servings: 4 to 6

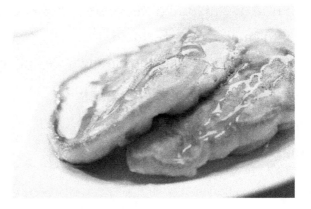

Ingredients:

- ¼ cup plain gelatin
- ¼ cup warm water
- 1 (14-ounce) can coconut milk
- ¾ cups coconut flour, sifted
- 2 tablespoons raw honey
- 1 teaspoon vanilla extract
- 1 ½ teaspoons baking powder
- ½ teaspoon salt

Instructions:

1. Whisk together the gelatin and water in a medium mixing bowl and let rest 2 minutes.
2. Whisk in the coconut milk, coconut flour, honey, vanilla, baking soda and salt.
3. Transfer the mixture to a blender and blend smooth.
4. Preheat a large nonstick skillet on medium-high heat and grease with cooking spray.
5. Spoon the batter into the pan, using about 2 to 3 tablespoons per pancake.
6. Cook for 1 to 2 minutes until bubbles form in the surface of the batter.
7. Flip the pancakes and cook for 1 to 2 minutes until the underside is browned.
8. Transfer the pancakes to a plate to keep warm and repeat with the remaining batter.

Fermented Coconut Yogurt

Servings: makes 4 cups

Ingredients:

- 2 glass pint-sized jars with lids
- 2 (14-ounce) cans coconut milk
- 2 teaspoons plain gelatin
- ¼ cup coconut milk yogurt (store-bought)
- Raw honey to taste

Instructions:

1. Preheat the oven to 100°F and fill a large stockpot about halfway with water.
2. Bring the water to boil then add the glass jars and simmer for 10 minutes to sterilize them.
3. Remove the jars and let them air dry.
4. Spoon the coconut milk into a medium saucepan then whisk smooth.
5. Sprinkle the gelatin over the coconut milk then bring it to a simmer on medium heat.
6. Whisk smooth then reduce heat and simmer for 6 to 10 minutes, stirring occasionally.
7. Remove from heat then let the mixture cool to 100°F.
8. Whisk in the coconut milk yogurt and honey then pour into jars and cover with the lids.
9. Place the jars in the oven and let rest for 12 to 24 hours then transfer to the refrigerator until thick.

Lunch Recipes

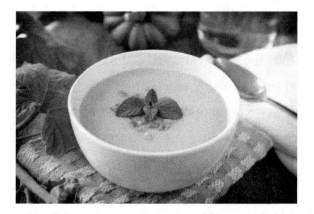

Roasted Acorn Squash Soup

Servings: 6

Ingredients:

- 2 large acorn squash
- Olive oil, as needed
- 1 tablespoon coconut oil
- 1 cup diced yellow onion
- 2 teaspoons fresh grated ginger
- 1 teaspoon minced garlic
- 2 teaspoons curry powder
- 1 teaspoon dried sage
- 3 cups low-sodium chicken broth
- Salt and pepper to taste

- 1 cup canned coconut milk

Instructions:

1. Preheat the oven to 350°F.
2. Cut the acorn squash in half and scoop out the seeds then discard them.
3. Place the squash upright on a baking sheet and brush with olive oil.
4. Roast for 35 to 40 minutes until the squash is fork-tender then remove from the oven and cool slightly.
5. Heat the coconut oil in a large saucepan over medium-high heat.
6. Add the onions, garlic and ginger then cook for 5 to 6 minutes until tender.
7. Stir in the curry powder and sage then cook for another minutes until fragrant.
8. Skin the squash and chop the flesh then stir it into the saucepan along with the chicken broth.
9. Season with salt and pepper to taste then bring to a boil.
10. Reduce heat and simmer for 20 minutes then remove from heat.
11. Puree the soup using an immersion blender then whisk in the coconut milk.
12. Adjust seasonings to taste and serve hot.

Baked Coconut Chicken Tenders

Servings: 6

Ingredients:

- 2 pounds boneless, skinless chicken breasts
- Salt and pepper to taste
- 6 tablespoons canned coconut milk
- 3 tablespoons plain gelatin
- 3 tablespoons warm water
- 1 cup coconut flour
- 2 ¼ cups shredded unsweetened coconut

Instructions:

1. Preheat the oven to 400°F and line a baking sheet with parchment.
2. Sandwich the chicken breasts between two pieces of waxed paper and pound thin with a meat mallet.
3. Cut the chicken into strips about 1 inch wide and season with salt and pepper to taste.
4. Whisk together the coconut milk, gelatin and water in a medium bowl.
5. Place the coconut and coconut flour in two separate shallow dishes.
6. Dredge the chicken strips in the coconut flour then dip them in the coconut milk mixture.

7. Dip the strips in the shredded coconut, coating on all sides, then place them on the baking sheet.
8. Bake for 10 to 12 minutes until the coconut is browned and the chicken cooked through.

Arugula Salad with Apples

Servings: 4

Ingredients:

- 8 cups fresh arugula, rinsed well
- 1 large granny smith apple, sliced very thin
- 1 seedless cucumber, sliced thin
- ½ small red onion, sliced thin
- 4 tablespoons olive oil
- 3 tablespoons apple cider vinegar
- 2 tablespoons fresh lemon juice
- 1 tablespoon honey
- Salt and pepper to taste

Instructions:

1. Toss together the arugula, apple, cucumber and red onion in a large salad bowl.
2. Whisk together the remaining ingredients in a separate bowl.
3. Drizzle the salad with the dressing and toss to coat.
4. Divide the salad among four salad plates to serve.

Slow Cooker Pulled Pork

Servings: 4 to 6

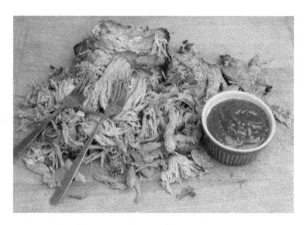

Ingredients:

- 2 large yellow onions, sliced
- 3 cloves minced garlic
- 2 pounds boneless pork shoulder
- Salt and pepper to taste
- 1 cup low-sodium beef broth
- ¼ cup raw honey
- 1 tablespoon coconut oil, melted
- 1 tablespoon red wine vinegar
- 2 teaspoons fresh lemon juice
- 1 ¼ teaspoon garlic powder
- 1 teaspoon ground ginger
- 1 cup diced shallots
- 1 cup fresh diced strawberries
- 1 cup diced carrots

Instructions:

1. Combine the onions and garlic in a slow cooker.
2. Season the pork with salt and pepper to taste then place it on top.
3. Pour in the broth then cover the slow cooker and cook on low heat for 8 hours until very tender.
4. Remove the pork to a cutting board and shred it with two forks before adding it back to the slow cooker.
5. Meanwhile, combine the remaining ingredients in a small saucepan and bring to a simmer.
6. Simmer for 20 minutes then transfer to a blender and blend smooth.
7. Pour the sauce into the slow cooker and stir it all together.
8. Cook on low heat for 30 minutes then serve hot.

Creamy Carrot Ginger Soup

Servings: 6

Ingredients:

- 1 tablespoon coconut oil
- 1 large yellow onion, chopped
- 1 inch fresh grated ginger
- 2 cloves minced garlic
- 1 large sweet potato, peeled and chopped
- 1 ½ pounds fresh carrots, sliced

- 6 cups low-sodium vegetable broth
- ½ cup canned coconut milk
- Salt and pepper to taste

Instructions:

1. Heat the coconut oil in a large saucepan over medium heat.
2. Add the onions, ginger and garlic then cook for 6 to 7 minutes until softened.
3. Stir in the sweet potatoes and carrots along with the broth.
4. Bring the mixture to a boil then reduce heat and simmer for 20 minutes.
5. Remove from heat and puree the soup in a high-speed blender.
6. Pour the soup back into the saucepan and whisk in the coconut milk.
7. Heat the soup until heated through then season with salt and pepper to taste.

Balsamic Chicken Salad

Servings: 4

Ingredients:

- ¼ cup balsamic vinegar
- 3 tablespoons olive oil

- 1 tablespoon raw honey
- 2 teaspoons minced garlic
- 1 ½ lbs. boneless chicken breast tenders
- Salt and pepper to taste
- 1 pounds fresh spinach, coarsely chopped
- 8 ounces sliced mushrooms
- ½ small red onion, sliced thin

Instructions:

1. Whisk together the balsamic vinegar, olive oil, honey and garlic in a small bowl.
2. Season the chicken with salt and pepper to taste then place it in a zippered freezer bag.
3. Pour in the marinade then shake to coat and chill for at least 1 hour.
4. Meanwhile, toss together the spinach, mushrooms and red onion in a large salad bowl.
5. Preheat the grill to medium-high heat and brush the grates with olive oil.
6. Place the chicken tenders on the grill perpendicular to the grates.
7. Cook for 2 minutes then flip and cook for another 2 minutes or until cooked through.
8. Slice the chicken and serve it on top of the salad with your choice of dressing.

Chilled Avocado Soup with Lime

Servings: 4 to 6

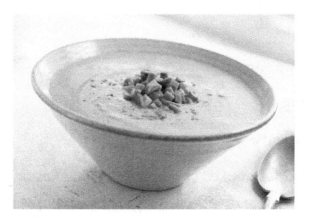

Ingredients:

- 2 large ripe avocado, pitted and chopped
- 1 bunch fresh chopped cilantro
- 1 tablespoon minced garlic
- 1 (14-ounce) can coconut milk
- 1 ¼ cups low-sodium vegetable broth
- 1/3 cup fresh lime juice
- Salt and pepper to taste

Instructions:

1. Place the avocado in a blender with the cilantro and garlic.
2. Pour in the broth, coconut milk and lime juice.
3. Blend the ingredients until smooth and well combined, adding water to thin if needed.

4. Season with salt and pepper to taste then pour into a bowl.
5. Cover the bowl with plastic and chill for 4 hours before serving.

Avocado Shrimp Salad

Servings: 4

Ingredients:

- 2 lbs. cooked shrimp, peeled and deveined
- 1 large ripe avocado, pitted and chopped
- 2 stalks celery, diced small
- ¼ cup fresh chopped parsley
- ½ cup canned coconut milk
- 4 tablespoons fresh lemon juice
- 2 green onions, sliced thin
- Salt and pepper to taste

Instructions:

1. If the shrimp is frozen, place it in a bowl of cold water and soak until thawed – you may need to replace the water once or twice.
2. Chop the shrimp coarsely and place it in a medium bowl.
3. Toss in the avocado, celery, and parsley.

4. In a small bowl, whisk together the remaining ingredients until smooth.
5. Toss the dressing with the shrimp, avocado, celery and parsley until evenly coated.
6. Chill the salad until ready to serve.

Dinner Recipes

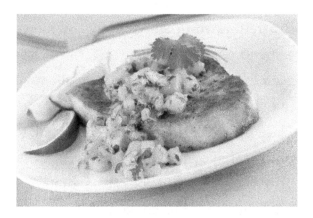

Seared Swordfish with Mango Salsa

Servings: 4

Ingredients:

- 4 (6-ounce) boneless swordfish steaks
- Olive oil, as needed
- Salt and pepper to taste
- 2 tablespoons coconut oil

- 1 ripe mango, pitted and diced
- ¼ cup diced red onion
- ¼ cup fresh chopped cilantro
- 1 tablespoon fresh lime juice
- 1 teaspoon raw honey

Instructions:

1. Preheat the oven to 400°F.
2. Brush the swordfish with olive oil then season with salt and pepper to taste.
3. Melt the coconut oil in a large skillet over medium-high heat.
4. Place the steaks in the skillet and cook for 3 minutes until seared on the underside.
5. Turn the steaks and cook for another 5 to 8 minutes until the fish is just cooked through.
6. Toss together the remaining ingredients in a bowl then spoon over the swordfish steaks to serve.

Rosemary Baked Chicken

Servings: 5 to 6

Ingredients:

- 1 tablespoon coconut oil
- 2 pounds bone-in chicken thighs and drumsticks
- Salt and pepper to taste

- 2 medium yellow onions, sliced thick
- 2 large carrots, sliced
- 1 cup fresh chopped broccoli fillets
- ¼ cup low-sodium chicken broth
- 2 tablespoons fresh chopped rosemary
- 1 tablespoon fresh chopped thyme

Instructions:

1. Preheat the oven to 400°F.
2. Heat the coconut oil in a large skillet over medium-high heat.
3. Season the chicken with salt and pepper to taste then add to the skillet.
4. Cook the chicken for 2 to 3 minutes on each side until browned.
5. Spread the onions, carrots, and broccoli in a rectangular glass baking sheet and drizzle with broth.
6. Place the chicken on top of the vegetables then sprinkle with rosemary and thyme.
7. Roast for 30 minutes then turn the chicken and roast for another 25 to 30 minutes until the juices run clear.

Garlic Herb Pork Loin

Servings: 6

Ingredients:

- 2 (1 ½ pounds) boneless pork tenderloins
- Salt and pepper to taste
- 2 tablespoons fresh minced garlic
- 2 tablespoons fresh chopped rosemary
- 1 tablespoon fresh chopped thyme
- 2 teaspoons fresh chopped oregano
- 1 teaspoon fresh chopped basil
- 3 to 4 tablespoons olive oil

Instructions:

1. Preheat the oven to 475°F and line a roasting pan with foil.
2. Season the pork with salt and pepper to taste then place them on the roasting pan.
3. Combine the remaining ingredients in a food processor and pulse into a paste.
4. Spread the paste over the pork then bake for 10 minutes.
5. Turn the tenderloins over then bake for another 8 to 10 minutes until the internal temperature reaches 155°F.

6. Transfer the tenderloins to a cutting board and let rest for 10 minutes before slicing.

Garlic Steamed Mussels

Servings: 6 to 8

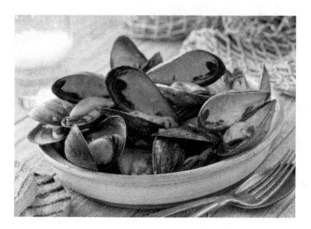

Ingredients:

- 4 pounds fresh mussels
- 2 tablespoons coconut oil
- 1 medium yellow onion, diced
- 2 tablespoons fresh minced garlic

Instructions:

1. Wash the mussels well with cool water, discarding any that are broken or that will not close.
2. Heat the coconut oil in a large stockpot on medium heat.

3. Stir in the onions and garlic then cook for 5 to 6 minutes until tender.
4. Add the mussels then pour in the broth.
5. Cover the pot and cook on high heat for 2 minutes.
6. Uncover the pot and stir the mussels then cook for another 3 to 4 minutes, covered, until the mussels have opened.
7. Spoon the mussels into bowls with the broth to serve.

Honey Grilled Salmon Fillets

Servings: 4

Ingredients:

- 4 (6-ounce) boneless, skinless salmon fillets
- Olive oil, as needed
- Salt and pepper to taste
- Raw honey, as needed

Instructions:

1. Preheat the grill to high heat and brush the grates with olive oil.
2. Brush the fillets with olive oil and season with salt and pepper to taste.
3. Place the fillets on the grill then close the lid and cook for 2 minutes.
4. Brush the fillets with honey then flip them.

5. Grill the fillets for another 3 to 5 minutes until just cooked through.

6. Brush the fillets with honey before serving.

Beef and Mushroom Stew

Servings: 6

Ingredients:

- 2 tablespoons coconut oil
- 1 ½ pounds grass-fed beef sirloin, fat trimmed
- Salt and pepper to taste
- 1 ½ cups low-sodium beef broth, divided
- 1 (14-ounce) can coconut milk
- 10 ounces sliced mushrooms

Instructions:

1. Melt the coconut oil in a large skillet over medium-high heat.

2. Season the beef with salt and pepper then add it to the hot skillet.

3. Cook for 1 to 2 minutes until the beef is browned then turn it and cook until browned on the other side.

4. Remove the beef to a plate with a slotted spoon.

5. Reheat the skillet then add the onions and garlic – cook for 5 to 6 minutes until softened.

6. Pour in ¼ cup broth and stir while cooking to loosen the browned bits.
7. Stir in the remaining broth and the coconut milk and cook until thick.
8. Add the mushrooms and beef back to the skillet and simmer for 5 to 10 minutes until the sauce is thick.

Seared Scallops with Caramelized Onions

Servings: 4

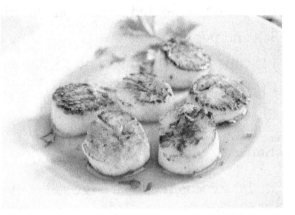

Ingredients:

- 2 tablespoons coconut oil
- 2 medium onions, sliced thin
- Salt and pepper to taste
- 1 lbs. large sea scallops, uncooked

Instructions:

1. Melt the coconut oil in a large skillet over medium heat.
2. Add the onions and season with salt and pepper to taste.
3. Cook the onions for 12 to 15 minutes, stirring occasionally, until caramelized.
4. Rinse the scallops in cool water then pat dry and season with salt and pepper to taste.
5. Push the onions to the side of the skillet then place the scallops in the middle.
6. Cook the scallops for 3 minutes then flip them.
7. Let the scallops cook for another 3 to 4 minutes until just cooked through. Serve hot with onions.

Lemon Artichoke Zucchini Pasta

Servings: 4

Ingredients:

- 1 tablespoon coconut oil
- 1 (14-ounce) can artichoke hearts, drained and chopped
- 1 medium yellow onion, chopped
- 2 cloves minced garlic
- 2 to 3 large zucchini
- 2 tablespoons fresh lemon juice
- Salt and pepper to taste

Instructions:

1. Heat the coconut oil in a large skillet over medium-high heat.
2. Add the artichokes, onions, and garlic then cook for 4 to 5 minutes until softened.
3. Peel the zucchini into noodle-like threads with a spiralizer or vegetable peeler.
4. Toss the zucchini noodles into the skillet with the lemon juice then season with salt and pepper to taste.
5. Cook the pasta for 1 to 2 minutes until heated through then serve hot.

Snack and Dessert Recipes

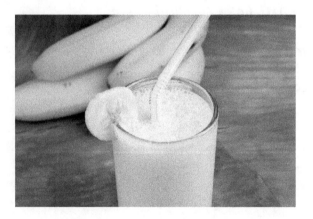

Cinnamon Banana Smoothie

Servings: 1 to 2

Ingredients:

- 2 small frozen bananas, peeled and chopped
- 1 cup canned coconut milk
- ½ cup ice cubes
- 1 teaspoon raw honey
- ½ teaspoon ground cinnamon

Instructions:

1. Combine all of the ingredients in a high-speed blender.
2. Pulse the ingredients several times to chop.
3. Blend on high speed for 30 to 60 seconds until the mixture is smooth and well combined.
4. Pour into a glass and enjoy immediately.

Coconut Apple Crisp

Servings: 6 to 8

Ingredients:

- 1 ½ lbs. apples, peeled, cored, and thinly sliced
- 2 tablespoons raw honey
- 1 tablespoon fresh lemon juice
- 1 ¼ teaspoon ground cinnamon
- 1 cup shredded unsweetened coconut
- 6 tablespoons coconut flour
- ½ cup melted coconut oil

- 1 ½ teaspoon vanilla extract

Instructions:

1. Preheat the oven to 350°F.
2. Place the apples in a large bowl then toss in the honey, lemon juice and cinnamon.
3. Spread the apples in a rectangular glass baking dish.
4. Combine the remaining ingredients in a separate bowl when spread over the apples.
5. Bake for 35 to 40 minutes until the top is brown and the apples are tender.
6. Cool the apple crisp for 10 minutes before serving.

Baked Squash Fries

Servings: 4

Ingredients:

- 1 large butternut squash
- 3 tablespoons olive oil
- Salt and pepper to taste

Instructions:

1. Preheat the oven to 425°F and line a baking sheet with parchment.
2. Cut the butternut squash in half then scoop out and discard the seeds.

3. Slice away the peel and cut the squash into sticks or wedges.
4. Toss the squash with olive oil, salt and pepper then spread on the baking sheet.
5. Bake for 20 to 25 minutes until golden brown and crisp.

Cucumber Melon Smoothie

Servings: 1 to 2

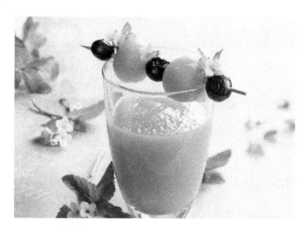

Ingredients:

- 1 ½ cups fresh chopped cantaloupe
- 1 small seedless cucumber, chopped
- 1 cup coconut water, chilled
- ½ cup canned coconut milk
- ½ cup ice cubes
- 1 teaspoon raw honey

Instructions:

1. Combine all of the ingredients in a high-speed blender.
2. Pulse the ingredients several times to chop.
3. Blend on high speed for 30 to 60 seconds until the mixture is smooth and well combined.
4. Pour into a glass and enjoy immediately.

Easy Coconut Flour Cookies

Servings: makes 2 dozen

Ingredients:

- 1 cup coconut flour, sifted
- ¾ cups coconut oil, room temperature
- 2 tablespoons raw honey
- 1 teaspoon vanilla extract

Instructions:

1. Preheat the oven to 350°F and line two cookie sheets with parchment.
2. Pour the coconut flour into a bowl and use a pastry blender to cut in the coconut oil.
3. Once you have a crumbled mixture, stir in the honey and vanilla extract to make a smooth dough.
4. Roll the dough into small 1-inch balls by hand and place them on the cookie sheets 2 inches apart.

5. Gently flatten the cookies with a fork then bake for 6 to 8 minutes until the edges are just browned.
6. Cool the cookies completely before serving.

Homemade Apple Fruit Leather

Servings: 4 to 6

Ingredients:

- 5 cups fresh chopped apples
- 2/3 cups water
- 2 to 3 tablespoons raw honey
- 1 tablespoon fresh lemon juice
- 2 teaspoons ground cinnamon

Instructions:

1. Combine the apples and water in a medium saucepan.
2. Bring the water to a simmer over medium heat then cover and cook for 12 to 15 minutes until tender.
3. Stir in the remaining ingredients then mash the apples with a potato masher.
4. Pour the mixture into a blender and blend smooth.
5. Line a rimmed baking sheet with parchment then spread the mixture on it in an even layer.
6. Bake for 2 to 3 hours at 170°F until tacky but no longer sticky.

7. Let the leather cool then cut into slices and roll them up in plastic wrap.

Vanilla Coconut Milk Ice Cream

Servings: makes 2 pints

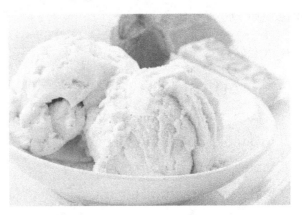

Ingredients:

- 2 (14-ounce) cans coconut milk
- ½ cup raw honey
- 1 tablespoon vanilla extract

Instructions:

1. Refrigerate the cans of coconut milk overnight then open them and spoon the contents into a large bowl.
2. Whisk the coconut milk until it is smooth then whisk in the honey to taste.
3. Once the desired level of sweetness is reached, whisk in the vanilla extract.

4. Spoon the mixture into a metal loaf pan and freeze solid.
5. When ready to serve, let the ice cream thaw ten minutes before scooping.

Salted Baked Zucchini Chips

Servings: 4

Ingredients:

- 2 large zucchini
- Salt, to taste
- Olive oil, as needed

Instructions:

1. Preheat the oven to 225°F and line a cookie sheet with parchment.
2. Use a mandolin to slice the zucchini as thin as possible then spread the slices out on paper towel.
3. Sprinkle the slices with salt and let rest for 10 minutes then blot dry.
4. Transfer the slices to the baking sheet and brush lightly with olive oil.
5. Sprinkle with salt then bake for 2 hours until crisp and dry.

Chapter Seven: Research

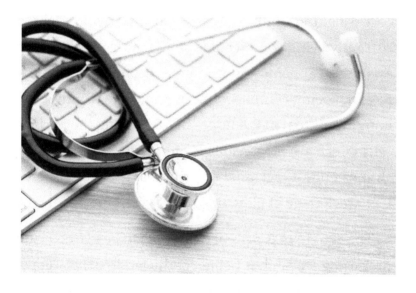

As is true for many autoimmune diseases, there is still a great deal to be learned about Guillain-Barré Syndrome. The medical and research community has made great bounds of progress since the initial description of the disease in the 1800s but there is more to be discovered. There are a number of research projects currently in the works, funded by such organizations as the National Institute of Neurological Disorders and Stroke and others. In this chapter you will receive an overview of the research being conducted regarding GBS as well as clinical trials that are current or in the works.

1. What Research is Being Conducted?

Most of the Guillain-Barré Syndrome research that is currently being conducted is aimed at two goals – refining existing treatments and finding new ones. There is also research being conducted in regard to the workings of the immune system in the hopes of identifying the particular cells which are responsible for initiating and facilitating the autoimmune attack on the peripheral nervous system which is characteristic of Guillain-Barré Syndrome.

Though there is a great deal more to be learned, some promising research is being conducted to delve deeper into the connection between Guillain-Barré Syndrome and certain bacterial or viral infections. Some discoveries have been made which suggest that there may be specific characteristics of some bacteria and viruses which activate the immune system in an inappropriate way, leading to an autoimmune response. It is possible that certain peptides and proteins found in bacteria and viruses may be the same as those found in the myelin sheath – if so, the production of antibodies to neutralize invading threats may actually trigger the attack on the protective myelin sheath which contributes to peripheral nervous system damage.

In order to make any true discoveries in regard to treatment options and a potential cure for Guillain-Barré

Syndrome, pharmacologists, immunologists, virologists, and neurological scientists must all work together. Guillain-Barré Syndrome is a very complex disorder, especially with its autoimmune component, so it may take time to make any real progress toward preventing and treating the disease more effectively.

2. Clinical Trials for Guillain-Barre Syndrome

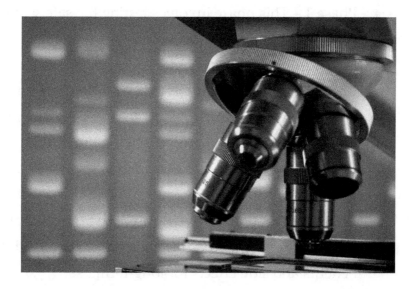

During the development of new therapies and treatments, testing is usually done on animal or insect subjects. When the testing is performed on human subjects it is called a "clinical trial". Clinical trials can be used to test different things but they all follow a specific order of steps and phases which are listed below:

- **Observational** – This phase involves testing the biomedical or health outcomes of the therapy in order to further understand the course of the disease.
- **Phase 0** – This phase involves testing the distribution of the new drug throughout the body at a very low dose – a dose that is below the therapeutic level.
- **Phase 1** – This phase involves testing the safety of the drug on a small group of people in order to determine the effective dosage.
- **Phase 2** – This phase involves testing the drug on a medium-sized group of people to determine its safety.
- **Phase 3** – This phase involves testing the drug on a larger group of people to determine its safety and to monitor side effects.
- **Phase 4** - This phase involves studying the drug after it has been marketed in order to further understand its benefits and side effects for long-term use.

Now that you understand how a clinical trial works, you may be curious to know what kind of clinical trials are in the works for Guillain-Barré Syndrome. Below you will find a brief overview of some of the clinical trials that are being conducted for this disease:

- *Inhibition of Complement Activation (Eculizumab) in Guillain-Barré Syndrome* (ICA-GBS), sponsored by the NHS Greater Glasgow and Clyde.

- *International Guillain-Barré Syndrome Outcome Study* (IGOS), sponsored by Erasmus Medical Center.
- *Can Exercise Reduce Disability in Peripheral Neuropathy*, sponsored by King's College London.
- *Second IVIg Dose in Guillain-Barré Syndrome Patients with Poor Prognosis*, sponsored by Erasmus Medical Center.
- *sCD163 as a Potential Biomarker in Guillain-Barré Syndrome*, sponsored by University of Aarhus.
- *The Changes of Cytokines in Guillain-Barré Syndrome: The Correlation with Clinical Manifestations and Skin Innervation*, sponsored by National Taiwan University Hospital.
- *Ultrasound in the Early Stages of Guillain-Barré Syndrome*, sponsored by Hans Berger Department of Neurology Jena University Hospital Friedrich-Schiller-University.
- *Prospective Study on Swallowing/Breathing Interactions in Severe Guillain-Barré Syndrome*, sponsored by Assistance Publique – Hopitaux de Paris.

- *Change of Nerve Conduction Properties in IVIg Dependent Neuropathies,* sponsored by University of Cologne.
- *Epidemiology Studies on Pediatric Guillain-Barré Syndrome, Fisher Syndrome, and Bickerstaff Brainstem Encephalitis,* sponsored by Chiba University Graduate School of Medicine.
- *Assessment of Chronic Guillain-Barré Syndrome Improvement with Use of 4-Aminopyridine,* sponsored by FDA Office of Orphan Products Development.
- *Study of Prevalence of Bladder Dysfunction and Urodynamic Findings in Guillain-Barré Syndrome; Their Correlation with Outcome,* sponsored by CSM Medical University Lucknow.

Chapter Eight: Frequently Asked Questions

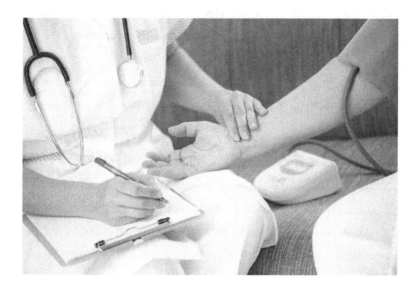

    After reading this book you should have a deeper understanding of what Guillain-Barré Syndrome and how it affects the human body. You have been introduced to the clinical signs and symptoms of the disease as well as the various subtypes and the typical progression of symptoms. You have also received information about the treatment options for Guillain-Barré Syndrome and research that is being conducted. Even after all of this, however, you may still have questions. This chapter is devoted to frequently asked questions about Guillain-Barré Syndrome and the Autoimmune Protocol.

Q: *How rare is Guillain-Barré Syndrome?*

A: This autoimmune condition affects roughly 1 out of 100,000 people in the United States. It affects people of all ages and does not affect men more than women.

Q: *Is Guillain-Barré Syndrome contagious?*

A: While it is true that the exact cause for Guillain-Barré Syndrome is unknown, it is clear that the disease is not contagious. There may be a genetic component Guillain-Barré Syndrome since it is an autoimmune disease, but just because a member of your family has an autoimmune disease does not guarantee that you will get one.

Q: *When should I see a doctor?*

A: If you are experiencing any symptoms of Guillain-Barré Syndrome you should see a doctor immediately. Though the disease typically progresses over the course of two to four weeks, it can progress in as little as 12 hours for some cases. Any symptoms of tingling, numbness, loss of sensation, or muscle weakness should be evaluated by a doctor immediately.

Q: *How long does it take to recover from Guillain-Barré Syndrome?*

A: Just as the progression of the disease is different for everyone, so is the rate of recovery. For some people recovery may occur over the course of a few days or weeks while, for others, it could take years. Even if you recover from Guillain-Barré Syndrome there is always the possibility for relapse or a flare-up of autoimmune symptoms.

Q: *Is Guillain-Barré Syndrome fatal?*

A: In some cases, Guillain-Barré Syndrome can be fatal if it causes respiratory failure or cardiac problems. As long as you seek treatment at the first sign of symptoms, however, the prognosis for this disease is generally good. Certain risk factors like old age and paralysis may make your outcome worse, so keep that in mind as well.

Q: *Can I eat dried fruit on the Autoimmune Protocol?*

A: It is best to avoid dried fruit because it is very high in fructose – you want to limit your fructose consumption to about 15 to 20 grams per day. That's about 2 servings of fresh fruit.

Q: *Why do I have to avoid nightshade vegetables?*

A: The term "nightshade" is used to categorize plants belonging to the Solanaceae family such as potatoes, eggplant, tomatoes, peppers and chilis. These are just the edible nightshades – most of them are poisonous. This should give you a clue as to why you shouldn't be eating nightshades but, more specifically, nightshades are bad for autoimmune disease because they interfere with the body's uptake and use of Vitamin D. As you have already learned, Vitamin D is very important for immunity.

Q: *What are "probiotic" foods?*

A: Probiotic foods are simply foods that contain live and active bacterial cultures. These are beneficial bacteria that help to balance the flora in your digestive tract, helping to support healthy digestion as well as immune system health (about 80% of your immune system is located in the gut). Some examples of probiotic foods include yogurt with active cultures and fermented foods like sauerkraut, kimchi, pickles, and kefir. For the AIP you can enjoy fermented foods, but avoid yogurt and other dairy products.

Q: *Which treatment option for Guillain-Barré Syndrome is the best choice for me?*

A: This is a question that only your doctor can answer. Guillain-Barré Syndrome affects different people in different ways so your treatment plan will have to be customized to the type of symptoms you are experiencing and the rate of progression for the disease. Most GBS patients respond well to immunoglobulin therapy and plasmapheresis, so your doctor is likely to prescribe one of these two treatment options.

Q: *Is there anything I can do to help with GBS research?*

A: If you want to donate money to support Guillain-Barré Syndrome research, contact the GBS/CIDP Foundation or the National Organization for Rare Disorders (NORD). You can find these organizations online at the following links:

<http://www.gbs-cidp.org/take-action/>

<http://rarediseases.org/advocate/>

Q: *Is a cure for Guillain-Barré Syndrome in the works?*

A: There is a great deal of research being conducted in regards to treatments for Guillain-Barré Syndrome including dozens of clinical trials. Unfortunately, no major discoveries have yet been made in regard to a cure for Guillain-Barré Syndrome or other autoimmune diseases but new treatments are always being found to provide relief from symptoms and to speed recovery.

Conclusion

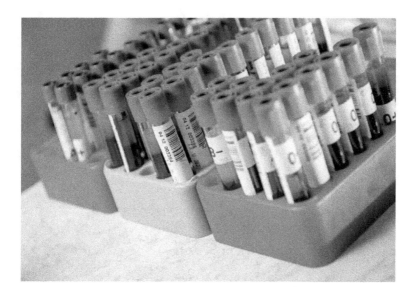

Whether you have Guillain-Barré Syndrome yourself or it is affecting a loved one, hopefully after reading this book you know that you are not alone. While this may be a serious and long-term condition, have hope in knowing that there are treatment options available and research is currently being conducted for refining those treatments and developing new ones. There may not be a cure for Guillain-Barré Syndrome yet, but someday there could be. Until then, use the information you learned in this book to treat and manage your condition with the help and support of your physician.

Index

H

I

L

leukocyte	9
lunch	55
lungs	10, 25

M

management	6
mechanism	21, 27
medical emergency	14, 42
medical history	35
medications	14, 40, 46
meningitis	35
Miller Fisher Syndrome	33
mobility	38, 40, 48, 49
motor	10, 13
muscles	9, 10, 22, 25, 30, 33, 35, 39, 48
myelin sheath	30, 31, 110

N

Nerve Conduction Study	35
nerves	9, 13, 25, 35, 39
nervous system	8, 9, 10, 13, 25
neurons	10, 13
nightshade	54, 118
numbness	17, 39, 117

O

onset	6, 21, 28, 33
organs	9, 12, 13, 19

P

R

References

"10 Signs You Have an Autoimmune Disease." Mind Body Green. <http://www.mindbodygreen.com/0-8843/10-signs-you-have-an-autoimmune-disease-how-to-reverse-it.html>

"All About Nightshades." Paleo Leap. <http://paleoleap.com/nightshades/>

"Autoimmune Disease." Healthline. <http://www.healthline.com/health/autoimmune-disorders#Overview1>

"Basics of Guillain-Barré Syndrome." Remedy's Health Communities. <http://www.healthcommunities.com/guillain-barre-syndrome/treatment.shtml

"Brain Maker Foods." Dr. Perlmutter. <http://www.drperlmutter.com/eat/brain-maker-foods/>

"Complications of Guillain-Barré Syndrome." NHS. <http://www.nhs.uk/conditions/guillain-barre-syndrome/Pages/complications.aspx>

"Dr. Weil's Anti-Inflammatory Diet." Dr. Weil. <http://www.drweil.com/drw/u/ART02012/anti-inflammatory-diet>

"Eat This: Probiotic Foods." Paleo Leap.
   <http://paleoleap.com/eat-probiotic-foods/>

"GBS Prognosis." Remedy's Health Communities.
   <http://www.healthcommunities.com/guillain-barre-
   syndrome/prognosis.shtml>

"Guillain-Barre Syndrome." Healthline.
   <http://www.healthline.com/health/guillain-barre-
   syndrome>

"Guillain-Barré Syndrome." Mayo Clinic. <http://www.
   mayoclinic.org/diseases-conditions/guillain-barre-
   syndrome/basics/definition/con-20025832>

"Guillain-Barre Syndrome – Clinical Trials." NHS.
   <http://www.nhs.uk/Conditions/Guillain-Barre-
   syndrome/Pages/clinical-trial.aspx?pn=6>

"Guillain-Barre Syndrome and Flu Vaccine." Centers for
   Disease Control and Prevention. <http://www.cdc.
   gov/flu/protect/vaccine/guillainbarre.htm>

"Guillain-Barre Syndrome Fact Sheet." National Institute of
   Neurological Disorders and Stroke. <http://www.ninds.
   nih.gov/disorders/gbs/detail_gbs.htm>

"Guillain-Barré Syndrome Treatment and Management."
   Medscape. <http://emedicine.medscape.com/article/
   315632-treatment>

"Organization of the Nervous System." <http://users.rcn.com/jkimball.ma.ultranet/BiologyPages/P/PNS.html>

Palmer, Sharon. "Is There a Link Between Nutrition and Autoimmune Disease?" Today's Dietician. <http://www.todaysdietitian.com/newarchives/110211p36.shtml>

"The Autoimmune Protocol." The Paleo Mom. <http://www.thepaleomom.com/autoimmunity/the-autoimmune-protocol>

"The Beginner's Guide to the Autoimmune Protocol." Ultimate Paleo Guide. <http://ultimatepaleoguide.com/autoimmune-protocol/>

"The Truth About Vitamin D: Vitamin D Food Sources." WebMD. <http://www.webmd.com/osteoporosis/features/the-truth-about-vitamin-d-vitamin-d-food-sources>

"What is AIP?" AIP Lifestyle. <https://aiplifestyle.com/>

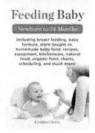

Feeding Baby
Cynthia Cherry
978-1941070000

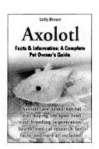

Axolotl
Lolly Brown
978-0989658430

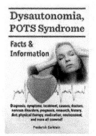

Dysautonomia, POTS
Syndrome
Frederick Earlstein
978-0989658485

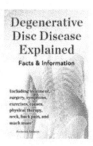

Degenerative Disc
Disease Explained
Frederick Earlstein
978-0989658485

Sinusitis, Hay Fever,
Allergic Rhinitis Explained
Frederick Earlstein
978-1941070024

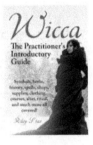

Wicca
Riley Star
978-1941070130

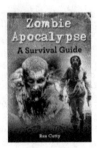

Zombie Apocalypse
Rex Cutty
978-1941070154

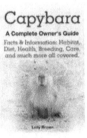

Capybara
Lolly Brown
978-1941070062

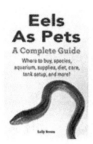

Eels As Pets
Lolly Brown
978-1941070167

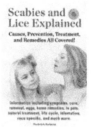

Scabies and Lice Explained
Frederick Earlstein
978-1941070017

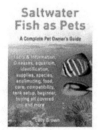

Saltwater Fish As Pets
Lolly Brown
978-0989658461

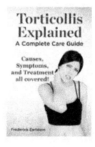

Torticollis Explained
Frederick Earlstein
978-1941070055

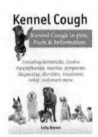

Kennel Cough
Lolly Brown
978-0989658409

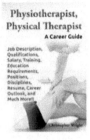

Physiotherapist, Physical
Therapist
Christopher Wright
978-0989658492

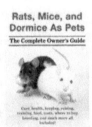

Rats, Mice, and Dormice
As Pets
Lolly Brown
978-1941070079

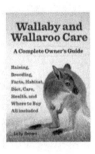

Wallaby and Wallaroo Care
Lolly Brown
978-1941070031

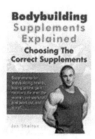

Bodybuilding Supplements
Explained
Jon Shelton
978-1941070239

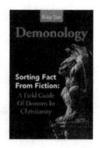

Demonology
Riley Star
978-19401070314

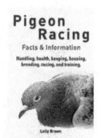

Pigeon Racing
Lolly Brown
978-1941070307

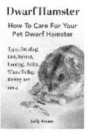

Dwarf Hamster
Lolly Brown
978-1941070390

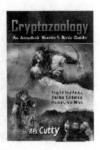

Cryptozoology
Rex Cutty
978-1941070406

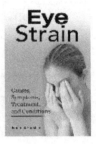

Eye Strain
Frederick Earlstein
978-1941070369

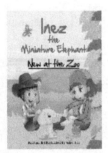

Inez The Miniature Elephant
Asher Ray
978-1941070353

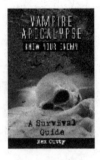

Vampire Apocalypse
Rex Cutty
978-1941070321